This book is part c
Heal Your Body, Cuit Your

ANXIETY, DEPRESSION, GRIEF, TRAUMA, PTSD, STRESS & BURNOUT

EMOTIONAL RELEASE, POSITIVE PSYCHOLOGY, MINDFULNESS, TAPPING, GRATITUDE & ENERGY MEDICINE FOR HAPPINESS & MENTAL HEALTH

DR. AMEET AGGARWAL ND.

ENJOY $35 & OTHER GIVEAWAYS

As a **Thank You** for purchasing my book, please enjoy **$35 off my online program** and other free giveaways on **health.drameet.com/p/freegift**

My online program covers a lot of what is in my book, plus:

How to regain energy you've lost to emotions, conflict & trauma

Using your 5 senses of sight, smell, taste, hearing and touch to heal emotions faster

How to improve weight loss by healing emotions, inflammation and adrenal fatigue

How I help people reduce their dependency on psychiatric medications

Special remedies for grief, loss, trauma and burnout

Expert interviews, including remedies to improve liver function

The program has even been approved for professional continuing education for naturopathic doctors, nutritionists & dietitians. Please visit health.drameet.com/p/freegift for your coupon and other giveaways.

Terms and conditions apply. Please visit website for more details.

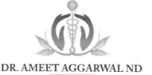

DR. AMEET AGGARWAL ND

Thank you!!

I dedicate this book to my beautiful mother, Kanta Devi Aggarwal.

Love you.

.

Acknowledgments

Thank you Trixie, Geeta, Shavika, Allison, Rubina, Steve, Paola, Marnee, Shelan, Anoma, Karen, Nita, Cheeko, Jess, Louisa and all my friends for making this book possible. Thank you Daniel of Dlight graphics for the illustrations. Thank you to my family for always being there for me. Thank you to the entire team of FIMAFRICA and all volunteers for your support and inspiration - I hope we can continue this amazing work. Thank you to all my patients for being with me on this journey and helping me learn so much from you. Thank you to all my teachers at the Canadian College of Naturopathic Medicine for inspiring me so much on this path of healing, and to my gestalt teachers for awakening my understanding of transforming consciousness. Transforming consciousness is a new path that we all must take, I believe, in order to uncover our strengths as well as our vulnerabilities, which is where our true power begins.

Table of Contents

Table of Contents of Dr. Ameet's Complete Book "Heal Your Body Cure Your Mind"

Preface

Who Am I, And Why Did I Write This Book?

I am a naturopathic doctor and practice a form of psychotherapy known as gestalt therapy. I help a lot of people with emotional problems through counseling and also by improving the health of their bodies. My job is both satisfying and frustrating because, as you've probably noticed, people with physical and emotional problems have a very tough time getting better.

Some take a lot of medicines or nutritional and herbal supplements and yet never resolve their emotional issues. Others go for counseling or read positive mindset books but never heal their bodies. This book shows you how to combine holistic medicine with positive thinking, since it is necessary to heal both your mind and body together in order to recover completely.

This book combines my personal experience and proven therapies I use with my patients to bring long-term relief from sadness, emotional pain, depression, anxiety, fear, irritability, stress, dissatisfaction, fatigue, and many other emotional issues. I have personally benefitted from these techniques and so have many of my patients who are now happier and emotionally stronger.

Even though the focus of this book is your emotional wellbeing, by following my advice you can resolve numerous other ailments, including digestive issues, hormonal problems, skin issues, obesity, asthma, joint problems, and other chronic diseases, since a large focus of this book is about reducing inflammation, stress and imbalance in your body – the major causes of most chronic diseases.

Here is what you will learn in this book and in Heal Your Body, Cure Your Mind.

Part 1 (This book) introduces different factors which affect your emotions. You'll learn how physical factors affect your emotional experiences. I'll show you how stressful experiences have a long term impact on emotional wellbeing and I give you powerful mental techniques to heal from stress and painful emotional experiences. You'll find out how to resolve turbulent emotions, change negative thoughts and beliefs, rewire your brain and develop more positive thoughts and habits to become more emotionally resilient and remain well for longer.

Part 2 (In Heal Your Body, Cure Your Mind) teaches you how your body affects your mind. I go into detail about your brain chemicals and how organs other than your brain play a key role in emotional wellbeing. This is something which doctors usually don't discuss or treat. You learn how diet, lifestyle and environmental toxins affect your body and mind, rendering you prone to recurrent bouts of emotional instability. You will learn to create balance throughout your body and heal the root cause of your emotional ill health using herbs, diet, lifestyle changes, yoga, breathing techniques and other powerful therapies. These therapies reduce the likelihood of you relapsing into emotional un-wellness. They reinforce your mental strength, build emotional resilience and help you remain healthy. You can read Part 2 before Part 1 or interchange between the two parts because it is vital to heal your mind and your body concurrently.

Part 3 (In Heal Your Body, Cure Your Mind) discusses how energy affects your mind and your body and why energetic healing, counseling and psychotherapy can be so important to your long term wellbeing. You will also understand how to use different homeopathic remedies, Bach flower remedies, nutritional supplements, acupuncture points and herbal remedies so that you can treat the root cause of your issues and remain healthy.

Even though I use the terms anxiety and depression liberally throughout this book, I have written it for anyone who wants to feel better. The advice in this book is useful for anyone who wants to be less stressed, heal from past stressful experiences, or just wants to feel more energized, healthy and positive. We all experience difficult situations in our lives that we need to heal from.

Unfortunately, surveys indicate that many people avoid seeking treatment or even refuse to admit that they have a problem because of the negative stigma associated with emotional problems. Some people think they will be judged as being weak or incapable of coping with life, not realizing that they have a very treatable condition that stems from very reasonable and non-shameful causes. Some people think their depressed emotions are part of their core personality and that they do not have emotional issues, so they do not seek help. Sadly, many of these people do not get help in time and let their life deteriorate further, sometimes even to the point of suicide.

It is not the goal of this book to replace medical advice. My goal is to help you treat the root cause of your emotional issues and resolve unfinished emotional experiences that contribute to your current emotional state, and to enable you to make healthier decisions for your road to wellbeing. I also hope that psychiatrists will read this book and look beyond mere medications to help people feel better. You might find that by using the techniques in this book you will require less medication. Please be responsible with your health and consult with a qualified professional before changing any of your medications or using some of the therapies described here.

You can find more remedies and therapies in my online program on health.drameet.com. At the time of writing this book, my online program has been approved for continuing education credits for dietitians, nutritionists and naturopathic doctors by professional bodies in different countries. I'd also like to offer you personal online sessions if you'd like more help with your health and emotions.

I wish you the best!

About The Author

Dr. Ameet Aggarwal ND was born in Nanyuki, a little town on the foothills of Mount Kenya, right on the equator. He travelled through various countries, touching the lives of many people through his intuitive understanding of deeper emotions. He graduated from The Canadian College of Naturopathic Medicine (CCNM), trained with The Gestalt Institute of Toronto and is also a Family Constellations therapist. He combines these therapies to provide the most comprehensive approach to mental and physical health - always aiming to treat the root cause, resolve emotional causes of disease and promote long term health.

After practicing in Canada, Ameet's passion for naturopathic medicine and homeopathy led him to start the charity The Foundation for Integrated Medicine in Africa (FIMAFRICA), and head to Kenya to provide naturopathic medicine to remote villages living without health care. He supervised and coached students and doctors from around the world who volunteered with FIMAFRICA, enhancing their clinical skills and personal development as human beings.

Dr. Ameet's therapy sessions, including online, are said to be some of the most profound transoformational therapies one can have. He is called to teach in different countries and works with different international organizations. His organizational work includes workplace wellness, conflict resolution, staff care, team building and burnout prevention.

His life transforming online program is even approved by various professional bodies as a continuing education course for naturopathic doctors, dietitians and nutritionists. You can join his free introductory video training on health.drameet.com.

PART I

Introduction

It is more important to know what sort of person has a disease than to know what sort of disease a person has.
~ Hippocrates (460– 377 B C)

"MY HEALTH WAS not the same as it was before, I could feel it. Even worse, my emotions were hitting rock bottom. I would lie in bed or on the floor, sometimes crying needlessly and feeling pity for myself. Crying would somehow bring me relief, but the gloominess never shifted. I didn't feel enthusiastic anymore. I had no motivation or confidence to do new things. My energy was not like it used to be. What I used to enjoy in the past didn't feel like so much fun anymore. Was there something wrong with me? What was wrong with me? What had changed me? I felt awkward talking to certain people because I thought they would not like me. I also felt guilty very easily. Why did I feel so guilty? I had to hide my tears sometimes when walking in the streets…tears of emotional pain for sometimes unknown reasons. Had someone told me I was depressed, I would have resisted, since I knew I was a stronger person, and in my opinion depressed people needed medications and I doubted I needed medication. I just had to figure out how to get out of this state…"

Get free videos and personal therapy on health.drameet.com

1

Do any of these feelings sound familiar to you? They might not. Even though I don't like to admit it, this was me, struggling with declining health and feelings of sadness, anxiety, and possible depression after a long stressful period in my life. Luckily, because of my training and tremendous help from my colleagues, I found my way out of this dark cloud. Using the techniques I have described in this book, I can truly say that I am much healthier and happier now; I feel more motivated, lighter, sure of myself; and I have much healthier personal relationships. I now even run training seminars, emotional healing and team building workshops and health retreats in exotic locations in Africa.

Factors That Effect Emotional Health

EVEN THOUGH I was struggling emotionally with a difficult situation in my life, I quickly realized it was not only external experiences that were affecting my wellbeing. The things I ate and my activity levels were strongly influencing my mental and physical health. I was very vulnerable to health issues, fatigue, anxiety and depressive thoughts. It was only after I started changing my diet and lifestyle, exercising and taking herbs and supplements that I began to realize the strong physiological connection with my emotions. My lifestyle habits were having a major impact on my body's chemistry and my body's chemistry was directly affecting my brain chemistry. I also worked with various therapists to release emotional experiences from my past, which were affecting the way I looked at the world and hindering me from enjoying my present life.

Because of my personal experience, my training, and experience with numerous patients, I really want you to look at the following areas of your life if you are struggling with health problems or your emotions and are trying to gain emotional peace and strength:

1. Has there been any physically or emotionally traumatic event in your life?

If there has been emotional trauma or stressful events in your life, the limbic part of your brain remains stressed even years after the trauma, and an unconscious part of you never fully recovers. You end up going through life permanently affected by the event. It becomes a part of your story. Therapies such as counseling, psychotherapy, homeopathic medicines, or Bach flower remedies, all of which I discuss in my complete book Heal Your Body, Cure Your Mind, help release emotional trauma from your conscious and unconscious mind and from your limbic brain. By releasing emotional trauma, you begin to experience life from a place of strength, liveliness, and authenticity.

2. Is a biological or chemical imbalance affecting your emotions?

Your mind is affected by neurotransmitters, hormones, and other chemical messengers floating around your body. Neurotransmitters and hormones are directly influenced by nutrients in the foods you eat, environmental toxins, and also by the health of your different organs. In *Heal Your Body, Cure Your Mind*, you will learn how your liver, adrenal glands, thyroid gland, and digestive system affect your mood. You will also learn how to heal these organs and use the right foods, nutrients, and herbs to correct the balance of your body. Doing this will enhance your wellbeing with long-lasting results, and reduce the ups and downs many people go through when they rely only on temporary fixes

3. Is there a stressful situation in your life or a lifestyle choice that is interfering with your ability to heal?

Chronic stress is the fastest way to break a person. Being around critical, aggressive, or emotionally abusive people keeps you in a perpetual state of stress. If you are in a stressful situation, whether socially or at work, you need to take immediate steps to move out of it or seek help to cope with it in a healthier and more empowered way. Equally, you need to exercise regularly to help your body recover from stress and learn to avoid certain unhealthy activities. Everyday activities that you may think are helping you relax can actually exacerbate your stress levels. Things like drinking too much alcohol or watching too much TV interfere with your chances of recovering fully. Abusing narcotic drugs, gossiping about others, talking negatively about life, hanging out with people who do not promote your wellbeing, spending too much time at work without caring for yourself, and doing things that do not help you feel good are also ways you stress your mind and your body without knowing it.

Unnecessary and unhealthy habits interfere with emotional healing and take up valuable time that could be spent improving your health. Try and fill every spare moment or idle time you have in the day with healthier activities, such as exercise, positive conversations, reading inspirational books, yoga, meditation, breathing exercises, and social activities that enhance your sense of wellbeing rather than make you sick and disappointed later on. In later chapters, I show you some easy feel-good exercises you can do to fill up your day and heal your emotions.

"Jane" was a thirty-four-year-old patient of mine suffering from chronic depression. She had been a volunteer in Somalia and had suffered stressful conflicts with her colleagues. She suffered from insomnia and binge eating as part of her depression. She had also suffered from chronic headaches since she was a child and had experienced her father being abusive toward her mother when she was growing up. The emotional trauma of her childhood had left her feeling vulnerable during conflicts, which led her to back away from standing up for herself as an adult and increased her stress at work.

In Jane's case, her emotional family history played a huge role in her susceptibility to fear and depression. At the same time, her chronic stress had depleted her adrenal glands, leaving her exhausted and unable to overcome emotional issues. In addition, her binge eating of a lot of starchy foods, combined with her stress, caused her blood-sugar, cortisol, and insulin levels to become unstable, leaving her exasperated and prone to chemical imbalances that affected her mood and her health. As part of Jane's healing journey, we encouraged her to eat healthy foods, which improved the level of brain chemicals in her blood. We resolved many of her previous emotional traumas using psychotherapy and energy based medicines such as homeopathy and Bach flower remedies, helping her to release the traumatic experiences that were still influencing her unconscious mind and affecting her behavior. We also built up her adrenal gland health using herbs and nutritional supplements so that her brain neurotransmitter levels corrected and stabilized for longer periods of time.

Jane's case was a typical case of depression that was resolved using a multi-angle, comprehensive holistic approach. She had to address her emotional history, her diet, as well as her physical health in order to feel emotionally well for longer periods of time.

The approach of resolving emotional experiences, restoring your body's optimal physical state and engaging in healthy daily activities is the cornerstone of building a foundation for emotional strength. By healing the root cause, you do not suppress symptoms, are less dependent on medication, and you will likely feel deeply better for much longer periods of time.

The Effects Of Emotional Experiences

All emotional experiences begin a physiological process in your body.
For every act, emotion, and expression of love, self-love, self-forgiveness,
and forgiveness toward another, your body reengages toward another
physiological process, closer to its original process, its healthiest process...
~ Dr. Ameet Aggarwal ND

EMOTIONAL AND TRAUMATIC events have a long-term impact on our health, be it a relationship breakup, parents fighting, divorces, a significant loss, financial difficulties, death of a loved one, or some other factor. Biologically speaking, your brain has the ability to create new neural connections based on what you experience. This ability is what doctors call **neuroplasticity**. Significant events alter the neural pathways in our brain, causing new nerve connections to be formed in order to cope with the stress and to anticipate similar events that may occur in the future. These new neural connections alter your perception of the world and of yourself so that things do not appear the same as they used to be when you were vibrant and happy. These new neural pathways also **alter the entire physiology of your body**, causing organs to function differently and causing chemicals, enzymes, and hormones to be made in different amounts, both of which directly affect your health and hinder your ability to recover emotionally.

Brain Connections Change Due to Neuroplasticity.

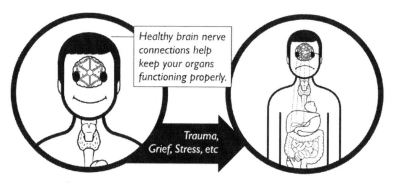

Healthy brain nerve connections help keep your organs functioning properly.

Trauma, Grief, Stress, etc

After stress and trauma, your brain develops unhealthy nerve connections to compensate for the stress. This has an unhealthy affect on your organs, causing emotional problems, certain diseases, changes in the way you see life and changes in behaviour.

Sometimes you might not even be aware that a particular emotional event has such a profound effect on you. If left unresolved or tucked away hidden under a stone in the back of your mind, the effects of these experiences continue to affect your mind and your body consciously, subconsciously, or unconsciously. This creates what I call **emotional holding patterns, or EHPs,** where your mind and body remain affected and continue to respond to emotional experiences as if they were still occurring, even though they might have finished. I believe that when the emotions surrounding your experience are too large for your mind to cope with, or if the EHPs go on for too long, a part of your mind shuts down and goes into depression. Depression is also partly due to a lack of trust in your environment based on previous stressful experiences and is also a state of exhaustion your body reaches when it can no longer cope with stress.

The chronic stress from EHPs taxes your stress-adapting organs such as your adrenal glands and thyroid glands. **Overstressed and under-functioning adrenal glands are a leading cause** of chronic anxiety, depression, and other health problems. You need to resolve or discharge EHPs in order to correct the altered neural pathways created in your brain, stop their negative effect on your body, and to give your brain a rest, rather than let it remain stressed from past events. Resolving stress and EHPs is also important because physically stressed organs in your body use up many more nutrients and produce more toxins than in a calm and relaxed body. When nutrients begin to run out in your body, your brain and other organs no longer have enough neurotransmitters and hormones to keep you happy and healthy.

"John" was thirty years old and had bipolar disorder, where he fluctuated between depression and manic or hyperactive and anxious states. The root cause of his condition was a traumatic divorce between his parents when he was seven years old and an unstable home environment while he was growing up. Because he experienced continuous stress as a young child, his whole development from childhood to adulthood was that of a stressed person. The constant threat and instability left his mind no way to feel safe, and he began to develop coping mechanisms that were dysfunctional to his body's natural rhythm.

John's treatment involved resolving the emotional pain from his memories using psychotherapy and homeopathic medicines and also stabilizing his adrenal glands, which were out of balance due to the chronic anxiety he grew up with *(I cover how to heal the body and use natural remedies in my book Heal Your Body, Cure Your Mind).*

With counseling, he realized how much stress he still carried due to his strained childhood. With counseling, he also developed the awareness and the power to deal with his anxiety and reconsider his adult surroundings with less stress and more peace. He felt safer trusting his external environment. After a few sessions of counseling and naturopathic medicine, John's condition resolved, and he had no more manic episodes. This was because he not only healed his body, but managed to resolve his emotional holding patterns.

Negative events from your past hinder your authentic expression and alter the way you interact with others. As you continue to live your life in a compensated way, you perpetuate the negative feelings you carry with you. Emotional healing is an opportunity to awaken the healthier and happier self within you and interact with others and with the world in a more positive way that inevitably gives you more positive experiences. As you recover emotionally from past events, you will begin to feel more confident and open in your life. With better health, you can gift yourself a more empowered and positive life.

Discharging and resolving stress and EHPs is possible through counseling, psychotherapy, talking to a friend, resolving the conflict and forgiving. Some of the best therapies I've experienced which release EHPs include gestalt therapy, emotional freedom technique (EFT), eye movement desensitization and reprocessing (EMDR, a type of psychotherapy), meditation and other mind healing exercises I teach you in this book.

Homeopathic medicines and Bach flower remedies, covered in my book *Heal Your Body, Cure Your Mind*, are energetic medicines that are also very effective in resolving EHPs. On the other hand, despite their efficacy and sometimes life enhancing benefits, I find that pharmaceutical medicines don't necessarily resolve EHPs – rather, they suppress symptoms and suppress your mind's ability to fully resolve difficult feelings.

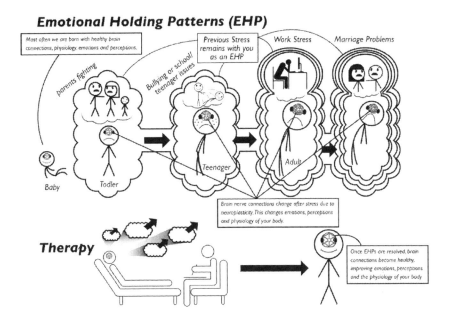

How Your Physical Body Affects Emotional Health

"To keep the body in good health is a duty...otherwise we shall not be able to keep our mind strong and clear."
~ Buddha

I SPENT A LOT of time going for psychotherapy and emotional healing with different therapists. It all worked reasonably well; however, there was always an underlying discomfort in my emotions. It was only when I started exercising regularly, treating myself with nutritional supplements and ate foods that were good for me that I began to see permanent results with my emotional strength.

Emotional *disease* is often due to an imbalance of chemicals (neurotransmitters) in your body and in your brain. Most people assume that emotional problems are due solely to chemical imbalances in the brain. Neurotransmitters, however, are produced and balanced by many organs in your body, not only your brain, and mood fluctuations are often a signal of something wrong happening with one of your other organs.

"Helen" came to see me with insomnia, anxiety, and painful and irregular menstrual periods. She was having too much sugar and drank three cups of coffee a day. The coffee was interfering with her liver function, which was affecting her sleep and her hormones (I teach you how to heal your liver and other organs for mental health in my book Heal Your Body, Cure Your Mind). The sugar and coffee were also reducing her *feel-good neurotransmitters* by ruining her adrenal glands and digestive system. Her lack of sleep was leaving her exhausted and making her anxiety worse. She ate very few vegetables, which starved her body of good nutrients and damaged her digestive system further, making her health even worse.

We changed her diet by removing coffee and sugar, and increased vegetables and protein-rich foods such as fish and chicken. We cleansed her liver using herbs and supplements. The results were astounding. Her menstrual periods became regular, her menstrual pains disappeared completely, her anxiety vanished, and healthy sleep patterns returned within three weeks. Not only that, her energy levels and concentration improved tremendously, and she was given a promotion at work. Her head-aches, which she hadn't brought to my attention, had also vanished. This is achieving optimal health. Improving your diet and restoring your organ health can have amazing benefits in your life.

"We must turn to nature itself, to the observations of the body in health and in disease to learn the truth."
~ Hippocrates

The organs apart from your brain that play an essential role in emotional stability are your *adrenal glands thyroid gland digestive system,* and *liver.* These organ systems are also crucial to the foundation of your overall health. Keeping them healthy prevents and treats many other diseases, including arthritis, hormonal imbalances, ovarian cysts, fibroids, asthma, eczema, digestive issues, and several other chronic health problems.

There are many factors that directly affect the health of all your organs and the levels of neurotransmitters in your body and therefore influence your emotions. Here are a few:

- Nutrient and vitamin deficiencies, such as vitamin B3, vitamin B6, vitamin B12, vitamin C, folic acid, zinc, essential fatty acids (EFAs), and other nutrients that affect mental health.

- Poor diets, such as too many simple carbohydrates and sugars or too little protein and vegetables.

- Insufficient nutrient absorption because of a malfunctioning digestive system.

- Food intolerances, allergies and inflammation.

- The amount of exercise you do. Regular exercise reduces depression and anxiety by increasing neurotransmitters in your body and increasing oxygenation of your brain and your organs.

- Blood-sugar balance. Unstable blood sugar often causes feelings of anxiety or depression, especially when not enough sugar feeds your brain.

- Hormonal imbalances caused by external estrogens, birth control pills, and water toxicity.

- Environmental and heavy metal toxicity such as lead, copper, mercury, aluminum, pesticides, and chemical toxicity.

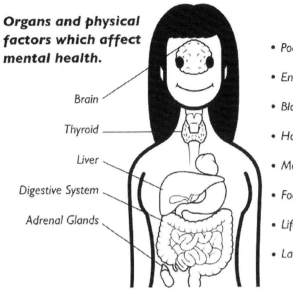

Organs and physical factors which affect mental health.

Brain

Thyroid

Liver

Digestive System

Adrenal Glands

- Poor diet and nutrition

- Environmental toxins

- Blood sugar imbalance

- Hormonal imbalance

- Medications

- Food allergies

- Lifestyle, late nights

- Lack of exercise

What Is Anxiety And Depression?

"Just like the unseen currents create winds, which you can feel, which move a leaf, which you can see, so do unseen thoughts create emotions, which you can feel, which create disease or healing, which you can see. We are all nature…"
~ Dr. Ameet Aggarwal ND

I DISLIKE USING THE word *depression* because it has such a heavy and permanent feel to it, and it comes with its own stigma. The word depression doesn't seem to help anyone get over their emotional state and sometimes makes people feel worse when they are labeled with it. I like to say it is not a *solution-oriented* label. Emotional *difficulty* is a better word because it feels more like a temporary situation, so I use it interchangeably with the words anxiety and depression.

Depression, anxiety, and other mental illnesses are diagnosed by doctors according to the *Diagnostic and Statistical Manual of Mental Disorders* (DSM-V). In this manual, different labels are given to different mental conditions, depending on the symptoms a person has and on the intensity and frequency of these symptoms. Labels given to people include *depression anxiety obsessive-compulsive disorder, major depression, seasonal affective disorder, generalized anxiety disorder, paranoia, bipolar, schizophrenia, post-traumatic stress disorder,* and others.

Similar symptoms do, of course, exist across different labels. For example, people with generalized anxiety disorder and major depression both experience symptoms of anxiety, although the frequency and intensity of symptoms in each label differ. Similarly, people with obsessive-compulsive disorder and generalized anxiety disorder both experience varying degrees of paranoia and anxiety, just in different amounts and with different resulting behaviors.

Even though different mental conditions are given different names, many of them share similar chemical imbalances. This similarity means that different mood disorders are actually similar processes occurring in the body with different triggers and different levels of intensity. This being said, try not to get emotionally attached to a diagnosis that a doctor might give you. The root cause, the affected organ system and your individuality are more relevant to your recovery. By knowing these important aspects, treatment becomes simpler and more effective.

In Jane's case it is important to realize that her symptoms of anxiety and depression are a result of her unique response to an abusive father and unstable home environment. Jane is different from any other person, so the way she responds to stress, diet, or environmental influences is different from how other people would react in similar circumstances. It is also vital to understand that other people with similar emotions to Jane might have a different cause to their emotions and need a different approach to their treatment.

For example, another patient of mine, Tina, thirty-three years old, had suffered from anxiety and depression since she was a child. No matter how much counseling she tried, she did not get better. We finally found out that she always got anxious and depressed after eating wheat. Her digestive system was intolerant to gluten, a substance found in wheat and other grains. The chemical reactions to gluten in her body were altering her brain chemistry, leading to her depression. After removing wheat from her diet, she recovered completely!

Symptoms of Depression and Anxiety

A person is diagnosed with depression typically when they have five of the symptoms below most of the time, persisting for longer than two weeks, and if these symptoms interfere with their social or work life. I believe many of us suffer with some of these symptoms enough to warrant healing, even though we might not be diagnosed with a mental illness.

- Excessive feelings of guilt, hopelessness, despair, and/or worthlessness.

- Difficulty concentrating or difficulty making decisions.

- Sleep disturbances—either insomnia or oversleeping.

- Unnecessary or chronic irritability.

- Avoiding social situations and activities or withdrawal from people.

- Fatigue or feeling tired often for no apparent reason. Lack of motivation, interest, or pleasure in activities they used to enjoy.

- Weeping frequently for no apparent reason, feeling sad all the time, gaining no pleasure from anything.

- Loss of or increased appetite or weight.

- Frequent thoughts of suicide.

Typical signs of anxiety include:

- Panic, restlessness, hyper-arousal, fear, paranoia, and intrusive or unwanted thoughts.

- Uncertainty, apprehension, indecision, hopelessness, or feeling paralyzed.

- Constant worry, tension, anxiousness, or uneasy feelings that have no definite explanation.

18

- Inability to feel confident about managing simple situations.

Sometimes depression and anxiety may manifest with physical signs, such as:

- Loose bowel movements, diarrhea, stomach cramps, or nausea

- Difficult or shallow breathing, tightness in the chest, heart palpitations, feelings of faintness, dizziness, dry mouth, or sweaty hands.

- Muscle pains, jaw tightness, grinding teeth at night or during the day, lack of sleep, or chronic fatigue.

Different situations that might cause anxiety in people include:

- Being in social gatherings.

- When a person is left alone and is uncomfortable being alone.

- When blood-sugar levels drop too low, due to physiological problems such as hypoglycemic episodes.

- When someone is confronted with their phobias; for example, failing an exam, meeting people, seeing a dog, or being exposed to heights.

- When someone is reminded of a traumatic experience that has not been fully resolved. This is most often seen in post-traumatic stress disorder (PTSD).

Different people respond differently to similar situations, which is why each person needs to be treated uniquely and individually. The way a person manifests his or her symptoms, be it anxiety, depression, or paranoia, depends on their unique characteristics, including genetics, diet, and physical and emotional makeup. A person's living conditions, work and social stress levels, support systems from people and community programs, socioeconomic status, and other factors also affect their ability to cope with stress and affect the way their emotions develop.

Mental Exercises To Improve Wellbeing & Heal The Past

"A man too busy to take care of his health is like a mechanic too busy to take care of his tools."
~ Spanish Proverb

A PRIMAL PART OF your brain, known as your limbic brain, is designed to protect you through instinctive survival mechanisms. Your limbic brain reacts automatically to situations based on previous stressful experiences you have had, and it can **continue to behave** in a defensive mode even though the initial threatening experience may no longer be present in your life. If a traumatic or stressful experience is not fully resolved, your brain will unconsciously continue to send stressful signals to your body, especially your adrenal glands. These signals put unnecessary and prolonged stress on your body, inevitably leading to adrenal fatigue, disease and emotional problems.

Psychotherapy, emotional freedom technique, homeopathic medicines, and other therapies that I describe below help free your brain from its unconscious stressed state and return it to its relaxed or neutral state, which also stops the stress your mind puts on your adrenal glands. Healing stressful emotional memories actually **changes unhealthy neural connections** in your brain into healthier connections, using neuroplasticity, which is the ability of your brain to rewire its nerve connections. Such changes actually alter the emotional interpretations you have of old stressful memories, allowing you to have more positive emotions and a longer lasting healthier perspective on life.

The exercises in this chapter help your brain resolve stressful situations from your past. They allow your brain to replace negative or stressful emotions with healthier emotions and thought patterns using neuroplasticity. This leaves you less traumatized and less stressed than before. As you do these exercises, remember to reduce inflammation and heal your body as well. **Inflammation and unbalanced hormones** actually **reduce the ability of your brain to make healthier nerve connections**, making it difficult to feel emotionally well even if you try and remain positive through these exercises. *My book Heal Your Body, Cure Your Mind covers healing inflammation, adrenal fatigue and hormonal issues in greater detail.*

Daily practice of the following exercises will reduce your predisposition to stress, anxiety, depression, and negative thoughts. Your mind will begin to feel safe. When your mind feels safe, you begin to relax and become more open to happier feelings. Having a positive and relaxed mind also helps you to expect more positive experiences in your life, which changes the way you approach life and brings better things to you. Your overall happiness will therefore be more a result of the **internal healing** of your own perceptions and emotions, rather than changes of external circumstances in your life.

Each of these exercises can be done separately or together, and some can be done every day. I highly suggest doing each and every exercise and doing the daily ones regularly. Try and do each exercise after reading it rather than going through them in your mind. If you fully engage in these exercises, you will experience more of their hidden benefits.

Healing the Past

These exercises help to release old and existing trauma from your mind so that you can free up your mind to become more present and enjoy life more fully. Try not to re-traumatize yourself when you think of some of your old memories – be gentle with yourself and seek professional help if some of these memories are too difficult to deal with on your own.

Timeline Release Healing Diary

Sometimes getting an overall perspective of our experiences in life helps to heal a lot of our beliefs and feelings. In this exercise, I'd like you to draw a timeline chart of your life, beginning from birth till your present life. You can use the chart I've drawn for you. On the left side, according to time, list all the physical experiences that had a significant impact on you. On the right side, list all the emotional experiences you have had in your life that either made you feel ashamed, traumatized, stressed, guilty, fearful, or unwanted, or created any other feeling that was uncomfortable. Even if you feel these experiences are irrelevant for you today, write them down still, because when they occurred, they did have an impact on you, however small. Also include some positive or happy experiences on the right hand side.

Now, starting with your most recent emotional experience that you can now safely write about, write continuously about anything that comes to mind surrounding this experience. **Write for fifteen minutes** without taking your pen off the paper. Continue writing even if what you're writing doesn't make sense.

This exercise helps you to **release trapped emotions** connected to your experiences and helps you to see your life more clearly and calmly. Do this for a maximum of two past experiences per day, not more, since you will not fully resolve the experiences if you crowd your mind with a lot of emotional processing.

You might need to repeat this exercise for certain events that take longer to resolve. Take your time in this healing journey. Be patient with yourself. Do not judge what you write on paper. Just continue writing over the next few weeks or months and notice how much better you feel as you get a renewed and more empowered perspective over your life.

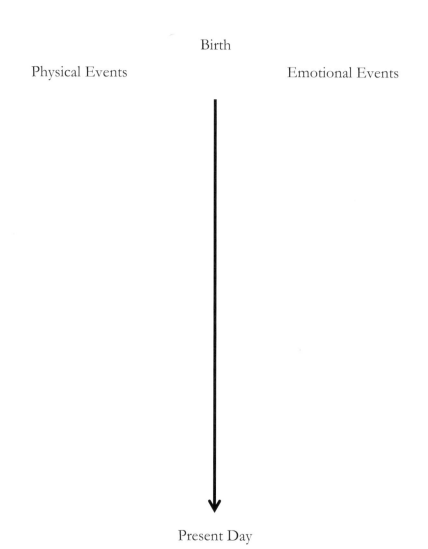

Birth

Physical Events   Emotional Events

Present Day

Forgiveness, Disappointments and Expectations

Forgiveness can be a difficult thing sometimes. Most of us, even when we try to forgive, are still left with a feeling of hurt or disappointment. This is normal. Even though you know it might be good for you to forgive someone or something, your mind might not be ready to let go or forget. In fact, sometimes saying *"I forgive you"* to someone still leaves you with a feeling that something wrong happened between you and that the person might still be guilty.

Through my training in family constellations therapy, I found a new humble and more complete way of saying "I forgive you". It's by saying "I'm sorry this happened for me with you", or "I'm sorry this happened for us", or "I'm sorry this happened for me with us", or a similar version to this. Saying it this way allows you to accept and let go of the situation more completely and peacefully. It also removes any blame you still hold for the person and doesn't leave you with a false sense of superiority. Try it out for some of the events from your timeline healing journal as well. Even if you don't feel like forgiving someone who hurt you or disappointed you, try saying this, either to them directly or in your mind, and see what happens.

Forgiveness sets your mind free of negative energy, thoughts and blame. It allows you to move forward more peacefully and positively.

Resentment and disappointment torment your mind, make you more negative and prevent you from living life positively. Similarly, unmet expectations can be a great source of unconscious depressive energy that we carry around with us. According to some therapists, unmet expectations and disappointments, especially related to our parents, can be a source of chronic depression without us knowing it. Think about all the unmet expectations or disappointments you have experienced with people or events. Whether you expected them to do something for you, or if they behaved in a certain way, or if they took something from you – whatever it is, do a mental check and see if you have any anger, resentment, disappointment or sad feelings around any memories. Do this for experiences from your timeline healing journal as well.

Now, really let go of these expectations and disappointments, and say the *forgiveness sentence "I'm sorry this happened..."* to all of these memories. Really make a mental effort to pull away from this stagnant energy which is holding you back from living life and smiling to yourself often enough. Say "It's safe to let go", or "It's safe to feel this way", or "It's safe to feel forgiveness sometimes", or any other sentence will free you from the grip of resentment and disappointment. Once you can move away from these feelings, your brain will rewire itself, and you will free up some mental space for more positive thoughts and feelings.

Emotional Freedom Technique

Developed by Gary Craig, Emotional Freedom Technique (EFT) is one of the fastest-growing methods people are using to find relief from emotional problems. In EFT, you **say statements** about your feelings and **tap on particular acupuncture points** on your body. Even though EFT may seem bizarre to do at first, EFT brings significant emotional relief immediately and changes negative beliefs and perceptions into more positive experiences.

- To perform EFT, choose an emotion or experience you are struggling with and that you want to change into a more positive one. You can also choose events from your timeline healing journal and heal some of the feelings and thoughts you had during those experiences. Doing EFT for past experiences rewires your brain and can heal hidden negative beliefs and feelings that you might not be aware of, but are still affecting you today.

- Using your right fingertips, tap on the fleshy part of the edge of your left palm below your little finger (known as the "karate chop point") while saying the following phrase three times: "Even though I... (Say your issue here, e.g., "am hurt by my partner's arrogance toward me" or "am feeling really depressed right now"), I deeply and completely love and accept and respect myself."

- Shorten your starting sentence into a summary sentence (for example, the above sentence can become, "hurt by Steven's arrogance"), and tap at least three times on the following points on your body while saying the shortened version of your sentence:

1. *On the bone near the inner corner of your eyebrow (left or right eye, it doesn't matter)*

2. *On the bone on the outer edge of your eye*

3. *On the bone underneath your eye*

4. *On the flesh above your lip and underneath your nose*

5. *On the flesh above your chin and beneath your lower lip*

6. *On the inner part of your collar bone*

7. *On your fourth rib underneath your breast*

8. *On the side of your ribs underneath your armpit*

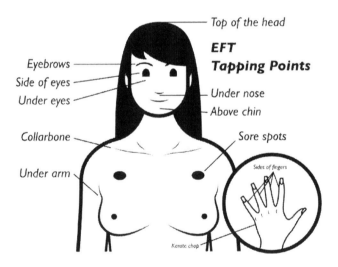

You might feel a shift in awareness about your feelings, and you can **alter your sentence to match your new feelings**. For example, you might say "less depressed" or "feeling relieved" while you continue to tap. Once you reach the end tapping point underneath your armpit, start again if you still have any negative feelings left. Change your sentence to closely match any new feelings you are experiencing. This is a simplified version of EFT and more details and more precise tapping points can be found on the internet, including free manuals on EFT. The beauty of EFT is that it uses acupuncture points as well as positive affirmations to create new neural connections in your brain, and it discharges emotional holding patterns, creating long-term benefits very easily.

Giving Yourself Permission to Heal

A lot of our emotional issues actually come from an unconscious resistance we have to allowing ourselves to accept a better way of being. Many of us are also **unwilling to let go** of certain ideas or emotions we have become used to. You might not even be aware of these subtle resistances which hold you back from feeling better. I have created an exercise which allows you to overcome some of these unconscious resistances. I used this exercise successfully when working with victims of the Kenya Westgate terrorist attack, and, even after such a traumatic experience, I saw people's anxiety peel away, their breathing change, and their trauma and tension turn to a sigh and smile of relief. It's a very powerful exercise if done right.

I'd like you to start a daily exercise where you say to yourself: "it's safe to (…be happy, feel this way, let go, heal, feel strong, feel hurt, be in love, etc….)" or "it's okay to …" and feel what happens inside of you as some of your limiting thoughts begin to surface.

This is a powerful exercise you can do for feelings connected to your past (timeline healing journal) and whenever you feel any emotional discomfort. I've used it many times and am always surprised to discover what thoughts have been holding me back without me even knowing it.

Whenever you try this exercise, search inside yourself for what you'd like to feel or what you're struggling with, and say "It's safe to…" Add the word "sometimes" or "once in a while" after your sentence. This helps your mind accept your sentences much more easily.

Even if you feel something negative and you don't know what belief is holding you back, try saying "It's safe to feel this way and recover" you'll suddenly give yourself permission to let go of your internal struggle and feel a sense of relief and internal strength. I'm listing a few sentences to help you on your way. Notice how you feel after saying each of these sentences. If you feel any resistance or emotion coming up, accept these feelings and allow them to change as you meditate deeper on your positive intention.

"It's safe (okay) to feel okay sometimes."

"It's safe (okay) to be happy again."

"It's safe (okay) to be rich and successful sometimes."

"It's safe (okay) to be okay with these feelings sometimes."

"It's safe (okay) to be in love again or to love someone again sometimes."

"It's safe (okay) to be in power again."

"It's safe (okay) to feel love for myself again once in a while."

"It's safe (okay) to feel this way sometimes."

"It's safe (okay) to smile to myself again once in a while."

"It's safe to feel important again, once in a while."

"It's safe to love myself again, once in a while."

Changing Your Story

In life, we often create a story for ourselves. For example, you might say things like, "I haven't recovered since my girlfriend broke up with me," or "I feel victimized by what happened, and it wasn't fair," or "I was too shy as a kid so I never made enough friends at school," or some other story that you keep identifying yourself with. If you identify yourself with what I call victimized or powerless stories, **you continuously behave as if these stories still have an effect on you**, and it becomes difficult to create healthier and more functional behaviors until you begin to change your story of yourself.

If you **retell your story** to yourself and to others in a different way, still keeping it truthful, you give your brain a chance to adjust and to feel a sense of power over the situation rather than feeling victimized. I tell you, this is one of the most powerful and life-changing exercises I have experienced.

For example, a small story from my childhood could be retold in the following way:

> My teacher walked up to me one day in the classroom and was very cross that I had my lunch box next to my desk. I had no idea that this was a problem. She picked it up and flung it across the floor to the other end of the classroom and screamed at me. I felt extreme shame and terror and have been afraid of her ever since.

I can slow down the events in my memory into different pieces, making it easier for my brain to process small parts of the story in little steps:

> I was sitting by my desk when suddenly my teacher walked up to my desk and was angry at me for something. I am not quite sure what. In her anger, she picked up my lunch box and threw it across the floor. I was ashamed and confused, and I think it was because my lunch box was next to me, even though I am still not sure if this was the real problem.

Since I have separated different parts of the experience into separate emotional components, I can see clearly that perhaps the teacher was not only angry with me, but just an angry person. I can even try a little humor in my story to make it lighter for me:

> My teacher was a really strict and angry woman, and all the kids were afraid of her. She even came up to me one day and threw my lunch box across the floor of the classroom and screamed at me. I was shocked, and all the kids were surprised, but we knew that was her typical behavior.

In retelling the story this time, I realize that a lot of kids were afraid of her and that maybe she was a generally angry woman. I give myself a chance to feel less guilt and shame about the whole situation because all the kids were afraid of her, and her anger was not only personalized toward me. I suddenly feel a sense of support from all the kids in the classroom. Perhaps my teacher did not know how to behave appropriately with children and was emotionally irresponsible. As I realize the generality of my teacher's anger, I feel a slight shift in my body where I was holding onto some fear from my past, and I now feel less threatened by the memory of her.

It might take many attempts for you to feel less emotionally affected by your story. This is OK. Every time you feel a slight shift in awareness or feeling, your brain is recovering from the event. You can also write your story out differently many times and go through the awareness shifts on your own; however, it's better to do it with people because of the energetic exchange you get from sharing with people. You can also do this as a group of about five or more people, with each person mingling with different people in the group, retelling their story in different ways with each person. Practice rewriting one of your memories, a couple of times, and see if it makes a difference to you.

Imagining Positive Experiences

Another exercise to resolve emotional trauma from an event is to imagine the event occurring on a stage or on a television screen, with you as a spectator in the audience. As you watch the experience, imagine the event occurring slightly differently. Use your mind to bring in helping scenes or more positive outcomes to the event.

For example, to heal myself of a situation when I was emotionally abused by someone in my past, I imagine him on the screen looking away briefly from me and being interested in something else. This lessens the intensity of his glare and actually helps me breathe a little more deeply. As I continue the exercise over time, I might be ready to imagine this person walking away periodically. This gives me more breathing space and helps my brain reprocess the event in a more relaxed way. Doing this repeatedly actually rewires your brain and alters your emotions surrounding stressful memories, therefore stopping your brain from continuously stressing your adrenal glands.

Another memory I healed this way is when I found it difficult to recover from the intense grief I went through during a prolonged breakup with my girlfriend. It was a long period of rejections and arguments where I suffered quite a bit. What I did to lessen the intensity of my grief was to imagine her on the screen smiling at me once in a while during our hard times. Doing this reduced the pain in my mind that was still there and helped me smile a little, too. You see, I didn't need to change the entire memory—I altered it subtly enough so it remained believable in my mind. As I continued this exercise, I actually resolved a lot of grief and self-esteem issues that stemmed from this event and managed to develop a healthy relationship with someone else.

A third example is the memory of a teacher who was really mean to me when I was a child. As I envision him on the screen glaring and shouting at the *little me*, I imagine a bird coming to rest on his shoulder. Automatically, this discharges the focus in my brain from his anger and menacing look to something more gentle and safe to experience for a young child. I might even imagine my parents or somebody larger coming to talk to him as a way of protecting me. This also reduces the anxiety in my unconscious memory. Because I am less threatened and feel safer emotionally with my memory, my brain stops sending stressful unconscious signals to my adrenal glands, and I regain some of my emotional strength.

You might initially feel intense emotions doing these exercises. As you continue to do them, the intensity will lessen because your brain will have discharged some of the stress associated with your memories. Negative events in your past hinder your authenticity and alter the way you behave with others. If you continue to live your life in a compensated way, you perpetuate the negative feelings you carry inside of you. As you recover emotionally from past events, you begin to feel more confident and open in your life. Healing is an opportunity to awaken a freer and more joyful self and to interact with the world in a more positive and self-supportive way, which will hopefully bring you better health and more positive experiences.

Ho' oponopono

Ho'oponopono is an ancient Hawaiian practice of forgiving and loving the part inside of you that is experiencing a trauma or disturbing event. Ho'oponopono became famous when Dr. Ihaleakala Hew Len in Hawaii cured mentally ill criminals without even seeing them. He would study their medical charts and look within himself to find which part of his consciousness created the person's illness in his reality. As he forgave and loved this part inside him, Dr. Len managed to cure a whole ward of patients.

This seems like a farfetched story, however it has worked for many people and is based on the principles that everyone's world is a projection of what's inside of them and we are responsible for everything we experience in our world. We can heal anything by taking full personal responsibility for the experience and healing the part in us that is creating the experience. To do Ho'oponopono, whenever you feel disturbed by a situation or have a past trauma that is not fully healed, allow yourself to open up to the part inside of you which feels hurt or troubled by the experience, whether it's in the past or in the present. Once you feel this place inside of you, place both hands over your heart area in the center of your chest and say the following words to this stressed part of you with as much love and compassion as possible:

"I'm sorry, I love you, I forgive you, thank you."

You can think of these words silently, whisper them or say them out loud. Keep saying them to the stressed part inside of you, notice how you feel and trust the changes you are feeling inside. Do Ho'oponopono on each experience you wrote in your timeline healing diary to help lessen the emotions surrounding difficult situations in your life. I do Ho'oponopono on daily situations and on many past experiences and I often notice a shift in my emotions, in the way I relate to people and in the way I behave now.

Relaxed Breath in Past Memories

This is an exercise I created and find that it works really well. If you have any memory that is stressful or negative, I invite you to reconnect with that memory in your mind. As you imagine yourself in that situation, notice how you are breathing. Begin calming your breath down, breathing in a relaxed way as you still focus on the memory. Allow your mind and emotions to shift as you continue to calm your breath down. Trust in the process and accept whatever changes are happening. Use this exercise on experiences you have written down in your timeline healing diary and notice how different you feel. Even though this seems like a very simple exercise, I find it very useful in helping our brain reorganize some of the disturbing memories that we carry.

Developing Emotional Resilience

The following exercises are things you can do daily to develop a positive mindset and better emotional resilience. Use them regularly, especially when you are going through difficult times, and watch out for change!

What Went Well the Previous Day

Research shows that remembering and writing down what went well for you during the day the increases your happiness for longer periods of time. I always do this exercise in the mornings in bed, especially when I used to wake up with that awful sense of dread, despair, and gloom. Remembering and writing down positive experiences helps your brain to better acknowledge that positive experiences are truly a part of your life and that not much has to change in your life for you to feel good every day. Writing and focusing on positive experiences every day also breaks your pattern of experiencing negative thoughts and beliefs, and you will eventually realize that you can feel good most of the time.

At the end of the day and every morning when you wake up, mentally go through or write down what you accomplished or what went well for you during the day and the previous day. It could be finishing a task, managing to exercise, going out with a friend, having a laugh, or even receiving a smile from someone. Make sure you acknowledge at least eight circumstances that went well for you or that made you happy. Try it now. Spend 20 minutes writing down everything that went well or did not go wrong for you for the past 2 days.

Being Grateful

I used to struggle with what *being grateful* means. I thought I was being grateful because I wasn't really criticizing anything in life. I thought that in the back of my mind I must already be grateful. However, after a few awakenings of realization in my life, I began to realize that being grateful is about fully and actively appreciating specific feelings and details about people, things or events. Being grateful involves a full hearted acknowledgment rather than something you think you already do in the back of your mind. Being grateful does not take away precious time from important things in life but actually gives you back important time to feel what's really precious in your life.

Being grateful is a powerful way to improve your emotional wellbeing. Studies show that people who practice gratitude are **less stressed and less depressed**. If you ever wake up in the morning with anxiety or a sense of dread, spend some moments feeling gratitude for as much as you can, and go through everything that went well for you, didn't go wrong or made you smile or relax the previous day. Every day write down ten things you are grateful for. When you wake up in the morning, say thank you for this wonderful day, and say thank you for at least five things you are or can be grateful for. Search your mind for people you could have thanked. If someone has been kind to you in the past, thank them verbally or in your mind if you cannot get a hold of them, even if it has been a while since you saw them last.

Instead of thinking about what is not going well in your life or what you still haven't accomplished, think about how much you wanted some of things you now have and acknowledge that they are now in your life, and appreciate it. Even in the most difficult circumstances, where nothing beneficial is apparent, find something you can be grateful for, even if it unrelated to the difficult situation. Searching for positive aspects of difficult situations **transforms the way you respond to life** and gives you the courage to be more proactive and create more positive changes for yourself. Practicing this regularly every day will infuse your mind with positive thoughts and emotions so you are less likely to lapse into negative feelings.

Make a **commitment** to yourself **for the next 7 days** to only imagine what is going well or what went well, doing this throughout the day for 7 days, no matter what is going on. If you're stressed or there's a stressful situation, pause for a moment, and divert your mind to think about what you are grateful for or what went well the previous day, or what has been going well for you in your life. It could be simple things like "I have a bed to sleep on", "I'm earning some money", "I'm grateful for my breath", or "I have a family or people who care about me". Over time your mind will automatically have more positive thoughts to think about, and will move away from stressful thoughts and painful emotions. Go ahead now and write about 10 things you can be grateful for.

Setting Positive Intentions

"To wish to be well is a part of becoming well." Seneca

Sometimes when we want change in our life, we focus too much on the negative thing we want to get rid of. Instead, talk about what you want in a positive way. State what you want, which gives your mind and heart a clear intention to work on, rather than saying what you want to get rid of, which is more complaining about your situation and reinforcing your negative thoughts and feelings. For example, rather than say, "I want to get rid of my sadness and depression," say words like, "I want to feel happier in my life." The second sentence increases the feeling of what you want in you, and it makes you more aware of the steps involved to get you to where you want to be. It also makes you aware of **certain feelings or ideas** that you have and were **not willing to give up on**. This clarity increases your ability to take the necessary steps to bring positive changes into your life. Write at least ten positive change sentences for yourself, and read them out loud at least once a day or whenever you're feeling gloomy.

Here are some positive change sentences that will help you get started:

- I want to feel calmer in my life (rather than saying, "I want to feel less anxious.")

- I want to smile more often.

- I want to have more positive thoughts

- I want to be and feel happy. I want to laugh more.

- I want to be in a relationship that is happy and good for me.

- I want to be in a place where I feel free and happy. I want to have positive thoughts about the future.

- I want to feel refreshed in the morning. I want to feel financially free.

- I want to be happier with myself; I want to think about myself and smile.

- I want to feel confident in myself. I want to heal from this.

Be specific about your goals and desires. Go ahead and write some down. Push yourself, explore, enjoy, and really feel the things you want! In the beginning, it might be difficult to pin down precisely what you want; however, as you do this process, a sense of clarity will emerge, and it will be easier to imagine what truly makes you feel better. After a while, you will automatically begin to let go of sadness, despair, and other negative thought patterns, and you will be able to focus more on positive thoughts and emotions.

Effective Meditations

"Nature, time and patience are three great physicians."
—H. G. Bohn

There was a time in my life when I was extremely stressed, confused and indecisive and had no sense of what I truly wanted for myself. I went to different therapists, and they all helped a bit, but nothing stopped the confusion or gave me a sense of peace until I started to meditate. As simple as it sounds, it was one of the most powerful gifts I gave myself. It helped me connect to an inner truth that really felt like my own, and this gave me so much power remain calm, make my own decisions and understand what I really wanted for myself.

Most people have their own specific way of meditating; however, some people find it quite difficult to meditate. I have described a few simple techniques for you below. Instead of trying to meditate for a long time at one sitting, it is actually more therapeutic to do **shorter meditations frequently during the day,** even for only five minutes at a time. Meditation helps you to develop more positive thoughts and make more rational decisions for yourself. Daily meditation improves neurotransmitter levels in your brain, reduces anxiety, lifts your mood, helps to resolve deeper emotional issues, and connects you to your higher spiritual self.

A simple meditation

- Sit in a comfortable position either on a cushion on the floor, or on a chair, with your back straight and the backs of your palms resting on your thighs.

- Touch the tips of your thumbs to your index fingers. Close your eyes softly, and shift your mind's focus to your breathing, allowing your breath to follow its natural rhythm.

- Imagine that your breath is made of white light and love, and all this light and love is **permeating every cell** of your body and healing every part of you wherever it goes, including your thoughts and emotions.

- Meditate in a calm, clean, and uncluttered environment, preferably close to some plants or out in nature. Share your healing light and love with the plants around you and imagine the plants sharing their healing light and love with you. This increases the amount of positive energy you receive from the environment.

- Meditate for at least two minutes whenever you have a chance during the day, and then slowly work your way up to ten minutes or longer.

- If your mind becomes crowded with thoughts during your meditation, observe these thoughts without trying to fight them away and without judging them. As you observe these thoughts, observe what reactions they evoke in you, and allow those reactions to occur without struggling against them. Let these thoughts disappear gently as you return to your visualization. Allowing your thoughts and feelings to come and go during your meditation develops harmony and patience in your mind and helps you become more comfortable and confident in yourself. As you become more comfortable with your feelings, your thoughts will have less power to create stress in your body.

- Other forms of meditation, apart from focusing on your breath, include visualizing different images, such as golden light in the center of your forehead, a peaceful candle flame, the ocean, the sky, or nature.

Another way to meditate is to visualize words like *joy, love, forgiveness, and peace.* **Smiling and meditating on positive words** can be very uplifting. Close your eyes and imagine the word *joy,* and let your feelings follow the idea of joy. Smile when you remember to smile and relax in the sensation of joy.

Meditating daily creates harmony in your heart, and you will feel less disturbed by stressful situations. Positivity will come more naturally to you, and you will begin to feel more comfortable with yourself.

Healing Rumination

"Sometimes your joy is the source of your smile, but sometimes your smile can be the source of your joy."
—*Thich Nhat Hanh*

Rumination happens when you spend time thinking negatively about your issues, self-reflect negatively, focus on feelings associated with negative situations in your life, or think about how you might have done things differently. Rumination often involves other thoughts such as fear, worry, regret, guilt, and shame, which re **not solution-oriented or forward-moving**. Rumination stresses your brain and makes anxiety and depression worse, and it also keeps you from engaging in healthier thoughts, conversations, relationships, and activities that would avoid negative feelings. The sad thing is that stressed, anxious, tired, and depressed people find it harder than others to stop rumination and turn their thoughts into more positive ones, making this a vicious cycle.

Rumination happens when your mind has not or cannot fully resolve a difficult emotional experience. Counseling, especially psychotherapy, reduces rumination by helping you come to terms with emotional experiences. By sharing your feelings with a therapist and releasing difficult emotions, your brain creates **new neural connections** that are **less emotionally charged.** . This healing allows you to feel happier and have healthier thoughts.

Rumination is sometimes hard to overcome because it involves thought processes that are trying to solve important issues in your life. Even if you want to stop, you might feel anxious about letting go of rumination because it means you will leave your problem unsolved and leave yourself vulnerable to the difficult situation. Feeling comfortable enough to let go of rumination and focus on other pleasant things will come with practice.

If counseling is not an option for you, there is another way to beat rumination. First, you need to recognize that rumination increases mental stress and depression and does not solve much. Second, think about the things you typically ruminate on and identify situations or times when you usually ruminate (like driving to work, sitting alone at home in the evenings, etc.). Catch yourself ruminating every time it happens, and **find a distraction** as soon as possible. Here are a few ways you can break the rumination cycle.

- Phone a friend, listen to some music, play with your pet, or go shopping and engage in conversations with the shop's staff or even with a stranger. If you can, share your feelings with a friend because it helps to get a different perspective on your problems and possible solutions.

- Do all the other exercises described in this chapter. Paint a picture or journal about your thoughts by writing continuously about them for five minutes straight without taking your pen off the paper. Free writing in this way releases emotions and creates healthier neural pathways in your brain. By resetting neural pathways, your brain loses some of its tendency to ruminate on the same memories because you have changed the emotional context of the memories through the emotional discharge.

- Start saying positive affirmations all the time. Positive affirmations break the cycle of negative thought patterns and also help you to begin believing that you can feel okay. Once you begin believing in more positive possibilities, your mind becomes more motivated and you end up feeling better more often. Say things to yourself like: "I'm happy, lucky, strong and blessed"; "good things happen to me every day"; "life is getting better and better for me every day"; "I feel good inside"; "It's okay to feel this way"; "I love you (to yourself in the mirror)"; "You're important (to yourself in the mirror)"; "sometimes these things happen and it's okay"; "it's okay to forgive myself sometimes". Even if you cannot believe or feel the essence of these sentences at the moment, continue saying them because by focusing on positive affirmations instead of negative ruminating thoughts, your brain actually feels less stressed and slowly begins to rewire itself towards better health.

- Do a quick set of sit-ups or push-ups; jog on the spot; clean the dishes; write down what you need to do for the week; go for a quick walk; or meditate on positive thoughts such as love, peace, and joy. I find exercise to be one of the best ways to break rumination, especially when I'm exercising with somebody else. Having company, even if you don't talk to each other, helps you engage with someone else rather than being preoccupied and isolated with your own thoughts.

- I avoid eating alone as much as possible. Eating alone can be extremely depressing. If you have to be alone while eating, listen to music or practice being grateful for every little thing in your life, including every bite of food. Studies show being grateful consistently minimizes the progression of depression. When I was visiting India, a hotel actually had a goldfish swimming in a bowl on every table occupied by single people.

- Do anything that is not thinking negatively about your issues, even if it means painting, smiling at the clouds, talking to a tree, or laughing at yourself.

Completing Small Tasks

Too often in depression we leave our life in shambles and allow unfinished activities to fester. A depressed person is not motivated to do much. The unfinished tasks linger in our minds and use up a lot of unconscious energy. We **lose energy this way**, and procrastination becomes both a habit and a struggle. The problem is, the more tasks you leave unfinished, the more overwhelming your life seems to be, discouraging you more from trying to accomplish anything and depressing you even further.

By accomplishing small tasks such as cleaning your bedroom, paying a bill, writing one email, or taking your dog for a walk, your mind actually **feels a sense of accomplishment**, satisfaction, and pleasure. Frequent experiences of accomplishment, pleasure, and satisfaction strengthen your sense of confidence and motivation, enabling you to do other tasks more easily. If you're feeling stuck, just trust that you have to complete one small task, and no matter how unmotivated you feel about it, commit yourself to completing it. Remember, it could be as small as mailing a letter, cleaning your room, paying a bill, writing your goals for the week (a really good activity), or calling someone you love. Once you start feeling the satisfaction of small accomplishments and recognize procrastination as the avoidance of risking change, you will feel motivated to do more for your life. Just start with one task at a time, right now!

Volunteering

Did you know that volunteering for a worthy cause actually improves emotional wellbeing? Yes, it's true. I've done it myself numerous times and it really feels good. Studies show that volunteering actually alleviates depression and prevents people from relapsing into depression as well. Volunteering also helps you develop social skills, gives you a chance to make contacts and friends, and prevents social isolation, which is a major cause and outcome of depression. Volunteering is often stress free and can feel rewarding, meaning your body will actually produce endorphins (feel good hormones) from feeling satisfied and appreciated. Give your time to a good cause this weekend, or whenever you have free time. Take a risk and find out what might be fun for you to do. You don't have to put yourself in a difficult situation to volunteer – I remember spending one weekend planting trees on Mount Kenya in the name of conservation. I'll give food to an orphanage for children with AIDS every Sunday, which is a really nice thing to do because the laughter and hugs from the children feels so good. These are just a couple of examples of nice environments where you can volunteer your time. And who knows, you might even help someone change their life for the better with a unique gift you didn't even realize you have!

Friends, Family, and Support Groups

"Friends are the medicine of life" - Unknown.

Being open with and gaining support from family, friends, and self-help groups can make a big difference if you suffer from emotional issues. It can be intimidating at first, but disclosing your problems to a trustworthy person starts a chain reaction of help and emotional release. They might give you advice, share a similar situation in their lives, or know someone who can help you. Even if you do not get all the help you need from the first person you talk to, sharing your problems with one person gives you the courage to open up and seek further help with other people.

As a friend or family member of someone with emotional issues, it is important to listen carefully when he or she discloses feelings and not be judgmental. Show that you care and are interested in the problems rather than immediately trying to suggest solutions. A person revealing anxieties and emotional issues is being vulnerable with you. The more you listen and allow that person to feel OK sharing this vulnerable side, the stronger and more open to help he or she will become.

Ask how you can be of help, but try to be patient and nonjudgmental if your help is refused. People with emotional difficulties often have a hard time judging the best solution. Another way you can help is to find meditation, yoga, personal-growth, or self-help groups. Perhaps you can attend a few sessions with the person to give some encouragement. Having support at the initial meeting or inquiry helps dissolve many barriers people experience when first seeking help.

ENJOY $35 & OTHER GIVEAWAYS

As a **Thank You** for purchasing my book, please enjoy **$35 off my online program** and other free giveaways on **health.drameet.com/p/freegift**

My online program covers a lot of what is in my book, plus:

How to regain energy you've lost to emotions, conflict & trauma

Using your 5 senses of sight, smell, taste, hearing and touch to heal emotions faster

How to improve weight loss by healing emotions, inflammation and adrenal fatigue

How I help people reduce their dependency on psychiatric medications

Special remedies for grief, loss, trauma and burnout

Expert interviews, including remedies to improve liver function

The program has even been approved for professional continuing education for naturopathic doctors, nutritionists & dietitians. Please visit health.drameet.com/p/freegift for your coupon and other giveaways.

Terms and conditions apply. Please visit website for more details.

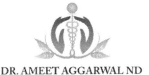

DR. AMEET AGGARWAL ND

Thank you!!

Summary

"Tears are often a sign of truth and not of weakness"
~ Dr. Ameet Aggarwal ND

We have covered a lot of ground in this book, and if you've read this far, now is a good time to go back over the sections that apply to you and start to implement the strategies that are most relevant to your circumstances. Here are some of the key points you should keep in mind as you do so.

To regain emotional strength, look at emotional or energetic areas of your life, including past experiences, physical issues in your body, and lifestyle factors that affect emotional health.

To resolve emotional experiences and energetic holding patterns, consider using:

- Bach flower remedies and homeopathic medicines

- Counseling, psychotherapy, or emotional freedom technique

- Acupuncture, Bowen therapy, or some other body therapy

- Meditation, positive visualization, and some of the other exercises described in this book to resolve emotional experiences

To treat your physical body, consider the following:

- Stabilize your adrenal glands using herbs, supplements, regular routines, healthy sleeping habits, and regular deep breathing techniques

- Heal your digestive system using herbs, probiotics and supplements and reduce inflammatory foods, drugs, and alcohol

- Detoxify your liver using herbs or supplements and eat lots of green vegetables and fiber to remove toxins from your digestive system.

- Eat correctly by minimizing sugars, avoiding junk food, eating nutritious foods, and ensuring you're eating enough protein

- Exercise or do yoga regularly to detoxify your body, increase oxygen flow to your tissues, stabilize your adrenal glands, and stabilize your brain chemicals

- Use physical therapies such as acupuncture, massage, or Bowen therapy, which have relaxing and other healthy benefits for your entire body.

I hope you gained something useful from this book. I think it is important to invest in yourself and live life enjoyably and as fully as you can make it. The more we can empower and help each other to do that, the better we will all feel.

If you like what you read in this book and would like a consultation, or have me work with your organization, please contact me through health.drameet.com. I wish you the best in life.

"It is health that is real wealth and not pieces of gold and silver."
—Mahatma Gandhi

Healing Through Inspiration And Transformational Awareness

PARADIGM SHIFTS ARE a way of looking at the world, situations, and your own personal experiences in a different way. They help you shift your perspective, behavior, and physiological response to the world inside and around you. I sometimes feel that a shift in perspective allows for change in our emotions, which inevitably brings about healing. I am including a few of my thoughts below to inspire you to allow changes in your emotions and in your life.

Healing is an aspect of letting go of perceived self so that true self may emerge free of disease.

All emotional experiences begin a physiological process in your body. For every act, emotion, and expression of love, self-love, self-forgiveness, and forgiveness toward another, your body reengages toward another physiological process, closer to its original process, its healthiest process...

Just like the unseen currents create winds, which you can feel, which move a leaf, which you can see, so do unseen thoughts create emotions, which you can feel, which create disease or healing, which you can see. We are all nature...

Accept, love and include every negative belief, thought and dark part of yourself as a full and integral part of your higher and lighter self because then it all begins to dissolve into the lighter higher conscious part of you; just like the way darkness in a room melts away when a candle is brought in... It can't be the other way around... Darkness does not put a candle out...

The Mathematics Of Disease

An experience creates a movement of energy. The movement of energy gains momentum, depending on the intensity of the experience. If left unhindered, the energy's momentum increases enough to create matter, which manifests as physical symptoms in your body. The longer you wait to intervene, the more work is required to reverse the momentum and undo disease. Very serious diseases and cellular degenerative diseases could be the momentum of energetic disease overcoming your body's resilience to recover itself from the intensity of the experience. By mentally engaging with and accepting the experience of the event that manifested the disease, we actually match our awareness to where the energy of the experience is, and time collapses so that the momentum of diseased energy dissolves into the present moment, thus freeing the mind and body from struggling against it and from manifesting symptoms.

If we didn't fully include ourselves in a difficult or stressful situation because we felt threatened or intimidated or something else, then we remain in a subconsciously stressed state, which alters our perception and behaviors. Until we realize the compensation, we create disease and disharmony in our lives.

Your vulnerability is from where your true power begins

Tears are often a sign of truth and not of weakness...

Allow yourself to succumb to yourself, for therein lies the peace and self-recognition.

The fear of change could be the fear of love…

Sometimes emotional pain is made up of the opinion you have of another person and their behavior. How many opinions do you hang on to? Let go and experience freedom.

Sometimes habit feels like intuition. It keeps you stuck in the familiar. It guides you to keep safe and avoid change. It doesn't necessarily bring what is best for you. Know the difference between guidance and intuition and habit and change…Step out of familiar and guidance and tolerate change till it becomes easy…

Procrastination could be the avoidance of risking change… Confidence comes more from doing not by not doing…

What entity is mind then, if it interferes with universal guidance?

A language engages our consciousness so that we think in a certain way. If we were to think in a different language, our consciousness would be different. If we would think in terms of in light and love, we would be free…

If your emotions are calm, the way you interpret your experiences will be calm. The same goes if your emotions are loving, peaceful, or any other way!

Bad habits occur when we become numb to the experiences that created them. Become aware…You have choice.

The advancement in medicine of the future will be love…

References

What is Anxiety and Depression?

- Strande, Alex, ND, PhD. September/October 2001. "Lifting Depression." *Awareness Magazine*. Accessed November 25th 2011 from http://www.simplyhealingclinic.com/articles/lifting_depression.html

How Your Physical Body Affects Emotional Health

- Morse, Trish. "Hormones affect anxiety and depression." Retrieved November 25th 2011 from http://www.hormone-jungle.com/depression.php.

- Pataracchia, Dr. Raymond J. BSc, ND. "Orthomolecular treatment for depression, anxiety, and behavior disorders." Accessed September 21, 2011 from http://www.nmrc.ca/pages/Nutritional_Treatment_of_Mental_Health.cfm.

- Mota-Pereira, J. "Moderate exercise improves depression parameters in treatment-resistant patients with major depressive disorder." *J Psychiatr Res*. August 11, 2011; 45(8): 1005-11. Accessed September 21, 2011. MEDLINE® is the source for the citation and abstract of this record.

- Hallberg, L. "Exercise-induced release of cytokines in patients with major depressive disorder." *J Affect Disord October* 1, 2010; 126(1-2): 262-7. Accessed September 21, 2011. MEDLINE® is the source for the citation and abstract of this record.

Mental Exercises to Improve Wellbeing and Heal The Past

- Seligman, M. Ph.D. Authentic Happiness: Using the New Positive Psychology to Realize Your Potential for Lasting Fulfillment. New York: The Free Press, 2002.

- Yook, K. "Intolerance of uncertainty, worry, and rumination in major depressive disorder and generalized anxiety disorder." *J Anxiety Disord.* August 1, 2010; 24(6): 623-8. MEDLINE® is the source for the citation and abstract of this record.

- The effects of rumination and negative cognitive styles on depression: a mediation analysis. Lo CS - *Behav Res Ther April* 1, 2008; 46(4): 487-95. Accessed September 21, 2011. MEDLINE® is the source for the citation and abstract of this record.

Made in the USA
San Bernardino, CA
01 July 2020